Glioblastoma Variations

Arias & Other Star Songs

By Greg Zeck

Dead White Man Press
Fayetteville, Arkansas
2024

ISBN 978-1-7356161-3-1

Manufactured in the United States of America

Cover art Jürgen Fälchle, Adobe Stock Photos

Typeset in 11-point Sitka Text and other Sitka styles

These poems are dedicated to Gerry, Teresa, Bob
— and all who suffer from brain cancer
both directly and empathically

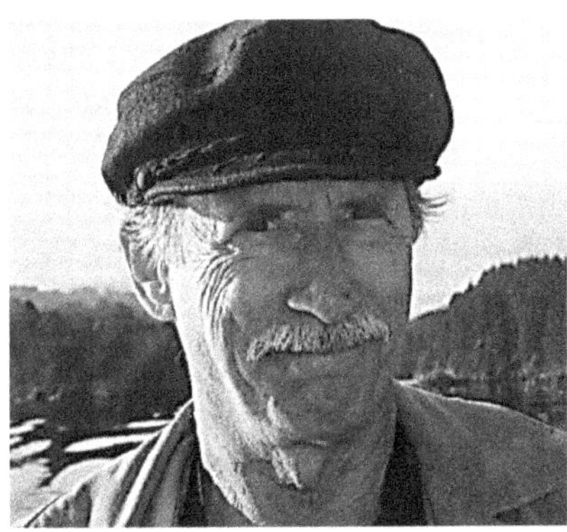

Gerald A. Zeck, 1939—2016

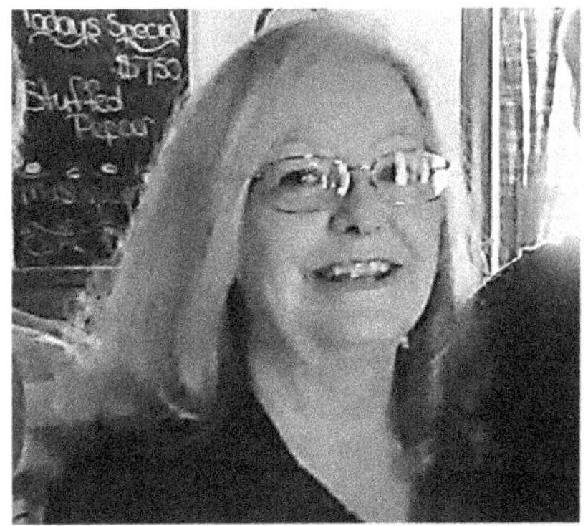

Teresa M. Phillipps, 1952—2022

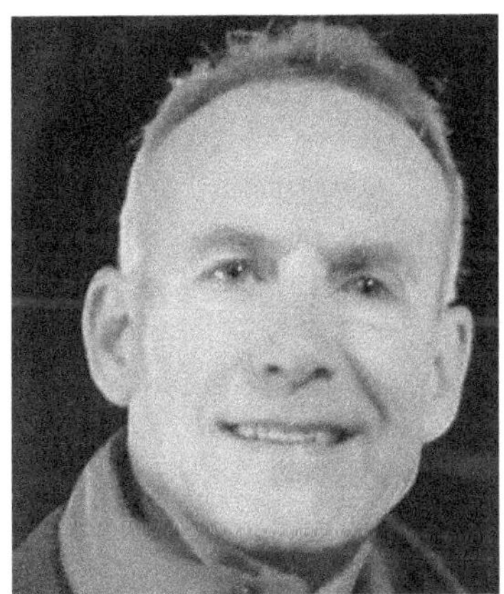

Robert T. Munger, 1958—2024

Epigraphs

"Every sentient creature suffers. When my self is no longer the all-consuming preoccupation it once was, when I see it as one narrative thread among myriad others, when I understand it to be as contingent and transient as anything else, then the barrier that separates 'me' from 'not me' begins to crumble … to embrace suffering culminates in greater empathy, the capacity to feel what it is like for the other to suffer, which is the ground for unsentimental compassion and love." — Stephen Batchelor, *Confessions of a Buddhist Atheist*[i] (see Endnotes, beginning p. 34, for this and all subsequent numbered notes)

"Of what is this house composed if not of the sun …"
— Wallace Stevens, "An Ordinary Evening in New Haven"[ii]

"The willows carried a slow sound,
A sarabande the wind mowed on the mead."
— Hart Crane, "Repose of Rivers"[iii]

Table of Contents

Prolog

The idea for this poem must have begun when my older brother, Gerry Zeck, who like many older brothers was a hero to his younger siblings, was diagnosed with glioblastoma, a nearly always fatal brain cancer, in June 2016. He lived less than four months after diagnosis and died on October 12, which used to be called Columbus Day and is now Indigenous Peoples' Day, a change that Gerry might have applauded, I think, given his fascination with the Mayans, whom he depicted in strange and wonderful line drawings, a few of which are included in this book.

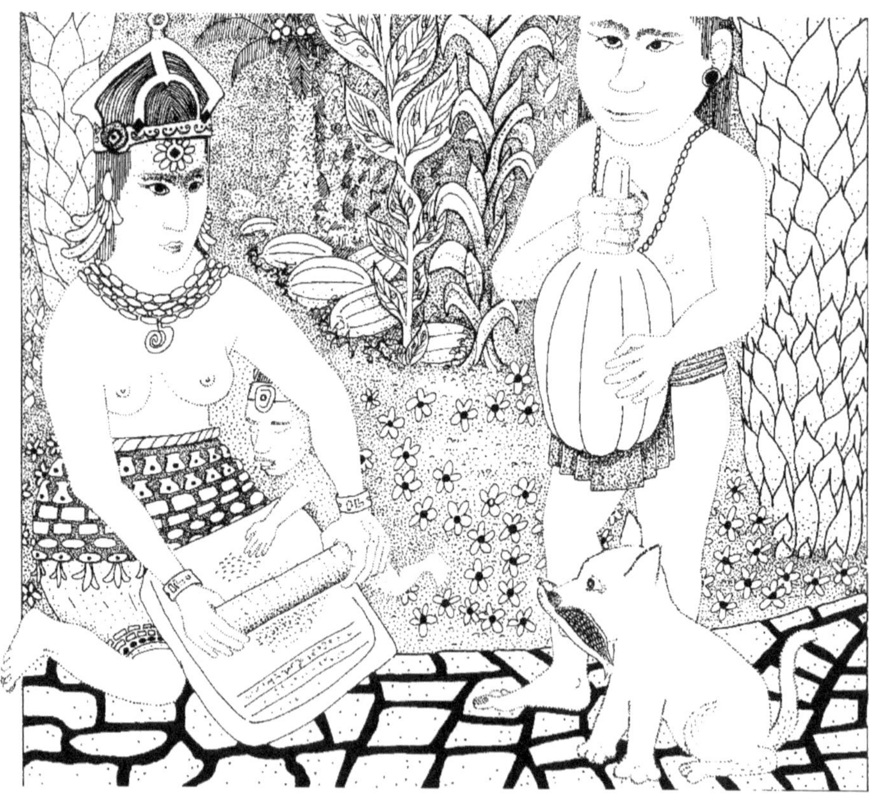

Gerry Zeck, Mayan Family, *1994*

A friend of my wife Jennifer and mine, Teresa Phillipps was diagnosed with the same fatal cancer in 2019, by which time she had moved back from Northwest Arkansas, where we met her, to her native New York state. An account of her affliction is given here, including the moment of discovery when she "went from calm / control to terror instantly" (III, 4:

individual poems are cited throughout by their Roman numeral first and then page number).

Teresa survived her diagnosis a year and a half, about average, about the same time that was granted our friend Bob Munger, the third subject of this short history of affliction, suffering, death, and wonder. Bob had been an architect and a designer of sustainable transportation projects; he was also a budding novelist. When Bob was diagnosed, he and his girlfriend, Tracey, took advantage of the latest options in healthcare and surgery, including the use of a device called Optune (IX, 11), but Bob too, like almost all others, succumbed to the inexorable progress of the disease.

So where does this sad story leave us? In the middle of life's dark wood, as Dante said? In a luminous space of our own devising? Bob Munger lost his eyesight after the third craniotomy and yet went on bravely every day he could. His was a fateful and infectious example, and it seems to me now that when Bob and I would go out together for ice cream (XV, 17) he was paying tribute to both the courage and the sweetness that life can offer even at its most dire. And was modeling how the rest of us might suffer, if suffering was inevitable, and the end was near.

To the Western mind perhaps, the Columbus view, it might be difficult to make out the sweetness in suffering and not to rebel or protest or sink into unutterable depression. Eastern and indigenous peoples, it could be, have a longer and less purely logical view of our contingence and transience (see Epigraphs, just before Table of Contents; Aria / Suffering, XIII, 15; and Aria / Theme & Glory, 33). And astronomers, too, whether Mayan or contemporary, may be able to move back from the infinitesimal scene of our suffering and appreciate how we human beings, in the vastness of space, might be seen, as Carl Sagan suggests, as mites circling a decaying plum.[iv]

The title and structure of this long poem occurred to me in a flash. I wasn't setting out, of course, to solve the mystery of brain cancer or even to console those who suffer. But the artistic example of J. S. Bach occurred to me, his great *Goldberg Variations* (1741), an aria plus 30 variations for harpsichord (now often played on piano), which came about, according to one account, when a Russian count brought with him to Leipzig a music pupil named Johann Gottlieb Goldberg

> … in order to have him given musical instruction by Bach. The Count was often ill and had sleepless nights. At such times, Goldberg, who lived in his house, had to spend the night in an antechamber, so as to play for him during his insomnia. ... Once the Count mentioned in Bach's presence that he would like to have some clavier pieces for Goldberg, which should be of such a smooth and somewhat lively character that he might be a little cheered up by them in his sleepless nights.[v]

The title page of the first publication suggests that the *Variations* are a "Keyboard exercise … Composed for connoisseurs for the refreshment of their spirits."

So a little cheer may be in order to refresh our spirits; to help us pass our sleepless nights and get past the bleakest of them; and to look out the window, from time to time, at the deep-sky objects (III, 4) aligned with the mystery of who we are and where we might be going.

Apology

A quick mea culpa, finally. I've cited a good number of technical-medical sources in the endnotes but cannot recall all my debts nor frankly think it worthwhile to acknowledge every last one of them as in an academic paper. You might surmise that some of my habits of mind are academic (I taught college English for a while, both writing and literature courses, and published academic papers); but few if any of my readers (of whom there may be few or any) will likely care much about strict academic probity. If any medical or technical scholar finds himself shortchanged here, he's welcome to apply to me for a share of the extravagant profits that I expect from this labor.

We should note that the technical-medical allusions here may soon be obsolete. In other words, current research and therapies may soon be superseded. Who knows? The cancer itself, some day, may be cured. But will be succeeded, we can be confident, by something else just as fatal. That's human, all too human. And so like life.

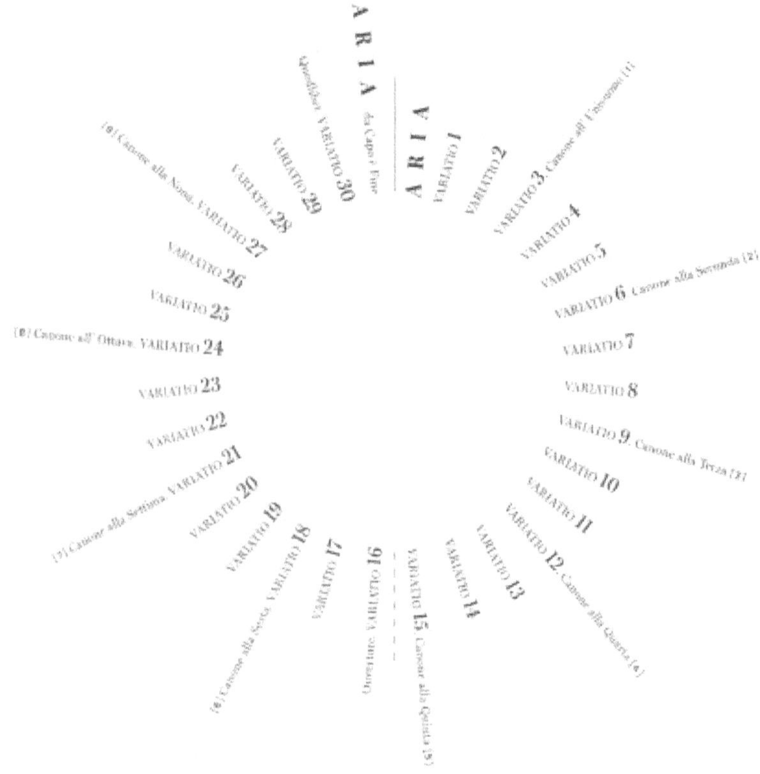

Structure of J. S. Bach's Goldberg Variations[vi]

Aria / Theme

It forms in the star
shaped cells of the brain
called astrocytes and multiplies
like malevolent loaves and fishes,
eating and eating away at the nervous
system. I would be nervous too, wouldn't
you, if so afflicted? Thank God, if there is a
God, or our lucky stars, if any, that it's our friends,
say ten years younger, or siblings, maybe ten years older,
or someone we wouldn't know from Adam or Eve suffering
a glioblastoma so that we ourselves, in some part of the brain,
or mind, I'm not a medical doctor and what do I know, or
philosopher, might be spared such suffering?[vii]

I. Arabesque / Etymophysiology

The ancient Greek *ástron,* or star, and *kútos,* cavity, give rise to astrocytes, the word, that is, not deed, and astrologia, the star words that talk to us in our hope and our despair, and astroglia, the star shaped glial cells that undergird the brain and spinal cord since the ancient Greeks and long before: glial, from Late Greek *glia,* glue, which may join us in argument, enjoin us, about the body and the soul and what is real and what is not. What kind of creatures would we be without brain and spinal cord and the semipermeable blood brain barrier of endothelial cells that helps keep pathogens out of the central nervous system (CNS)?

Or the words that make possible our course, our discourse? Our way out of the cave and its shadows? Moving our lips both to kiss and to love, to tell both time and truth?

Apologies here for the technical, the merely technical, yet what other recourse, resource do we have here at the beginning of the end, as the brain, the most delicate organ of the human body comes to mind, and so is bound up with what might be called both soul and reason?

Under our lucky stars, or not, magnetic resonance imaging (MRI) reveals instantly how the feet of the astrocyte lift up the brain, uplift it, keeping it from harm. That's the idea anyway. Imagine, because can we actually see them, these hidden and forbidding and essential things?

II. Allemande

Let's say this is a song, a dance, as it is song and dance
here on the page: a loose body posture: now, come,
friends, we dance a German dance that Bach himself
might have known, back in the day, hold hands
and come close, tantalizingly. Gather on the dance
floor of these verses even now, swaying, accentuating
our intentions as we come to know them. Gesture
with our hands, stepping here and there. Think upbeat,
in this lively allemande, of those in the best of health
as well as those sorely pressed by circumstance.
We live, brothers, sisters, and we dance.

Gather round, all you who thirst and hunger
for justice's sake. Shake a leg, extend your hands,
feel each other's pain. We are all family here, *nicht wahr?*[viii]

In this duple meter and moderate tempo, we bow,
one to the other. Grieving, hoping, we caste our eyes,
as divers colors as they are, toward each other
and the heavens too, seeking communion,
hoping for a glimpse through the scudding clouds,
the mumbling thunder, of the celestial blue.

III. Canon / Teresa and the Stars

One cold November morning, a few years ago,
sixty six behind her, the best time of the year
to observe deep sky objects, she went to the coffee
maker and couldn't figure out how to use the coffee
maker. Ditto with phone and computer. Was it
a stroke? She drove to the ER without problem,
looking up at the northern heavens, but once
there could not talk or write, and went from calm
control to terror instantly. The Andromeda Galaxy,
for example, the Wizard Nebula. That cold November
morning, then and now, when we might be glad
and guilty, the rest of us, that, for the time being,
all we have, the best time of our lives, we are spared?
A golfball size tumor in the brain was imaged, as much
as possible excised, and chemo rods implanted. Imagine
also the Heart and Soul Nebulae. In the sidereal scheme
of things, consider twelve to seventeen months par
for the course. Then too the Sculptor and Cartwheel
galaxies, Robert's Quartet, and the Magellanic Cloud.

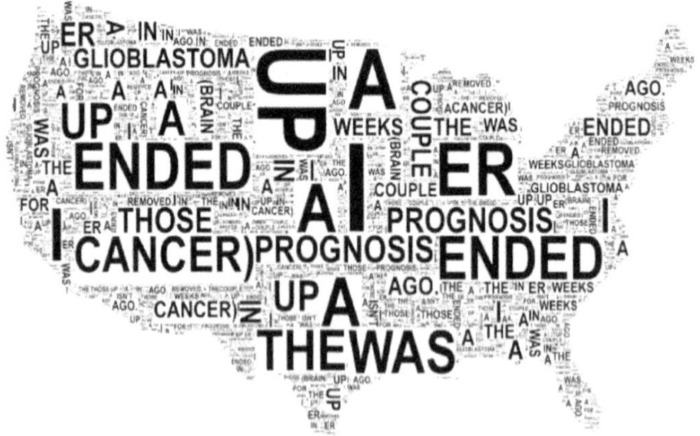

Teresa Phillipps, Facebook post on discovery of her glioblastoma,
12/1/2019. Graphic created via Wordificator.[ix]

IV. Dance / Varying Tempo

I can't help but think of crabs, their forms like stars,
like cancer, like nothing else. As the deck hand said,
wrangling aboard crab pots in stormy seas, just look
at the size of those bastards.[x] At least those bastards
were dead or were soon to be dead. Or in some wealthy
bastard's mouth, covered with butter and, say, tarragon,
someone not thinking of cancer or his half million dollar
income, someone with not a cure in the world.

V. Arabesque / Etymotechnical

Technical, from Greek *techne,* craft or art, related to the Proto Indo European *teks,* weave or fabricate, as in textile or text. I wouldn't be pulling your leg, would I, or making this stuff up whole cloth? The technical, the phenomenal are with us in this cave, this shit cave,[xi] pardon my French, it's a filthy language, before we exit, make a break for the noumenal, if we make a break at all or are simply broken. It's glias that cast these spells, turn malignant and spread: metastasize the word. It's glioblastoma multiforme (GBM), the most common primary brain tumor in adults, that remains at this date, the year of our Lord whatever the hell it is, if any, for many have no lord, it's true, and what does date matter, incurable, with a median survival rate of fifteen months according to one source. The cancer of time is eating us away[xii] even as we curse our fate, or the fate of those less fortunate than we, who might be called victims, discoursing on, cursing primary brain cancers, those that originate in the brain — and first manifest in a variety of ways, say difficulties speaking, hearing, seeing, grasping objects, controlling impulses, headaches, seizures, vomiting, nausea, numbness. We declare war against cancer. We get down in the dirt and blood and shit of the trenches, mobilizing against time, the first line of defense, where for better or worse there are no atheists and work this out, yes, work like hell to make our way out of this, to come out of this darkness into the blinding light.

VI. Canon / Gerald in God's Waiting Room

Late June a few years ago, my brother Gerry, eight
years older and perhaps entitled to a few geriatric
complications, was having trouble down in Florida,
God's waiting room he called it where he was waiting
and searching too. His girlfriend Lisa was puzzled,
the younger, hotter one for whom he left his wife
of forty five years, the one he was fucking on the sly,
and then when his wife Pam, who'd recovered
from breast cancer a few years before, a damn good
textile artist herself, found his texts to the GF and kicked
him out he found his girlfriend's house was not really
his house, surprise, and had plans to move out and find
a house, a mind of his own. He was helping the GF on
the turtle patrol, confused and newly hatched creatures
scrambling up the sand toward the luminous houses
of the rich, not the gulf that yawed and gulped and beckoned
behind them. Late June a few years ago, now and then,
that is, Gerseybro would drop the hatchlings from his hands,
and Lisa would say what's wrong with you and why are you
drooling? An artist, he had plans also for an artist's studio
where he might continue to pursue, in pen and ink,
the creature he called Tanda, his anima, shaped like a pen's
nib, penis, hard to know. He'd been taking testosterone,
at his age, getting hard, horny, hairy, and living at the same
time too much in his mind. He chased herm, we might say,
him or her, Tanda, to the end, not termination but telos,
from the Greek *télos,* end, purpose, or goal, for what is
man's end or object? Not simply to eat and shit and fuck
and die, is it, natural enough and material to this tale,
but produce something beyond it? But to actualize, pardon
the jargon, or realize a potential that's in us somehow,
someway, from the start, from the stars?

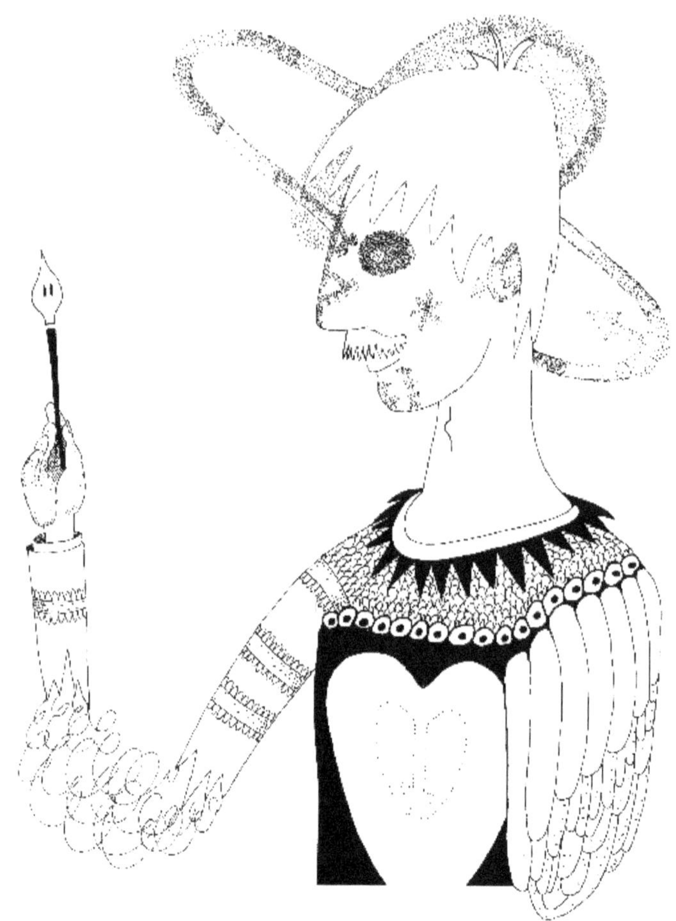

Gerry Zeck, Tanda Mirror, *1994*

VII. Dance / Reprise

So cancer is crab in Latin, and in astrology
a sign of feelings and the artistic soul.
So Dr. Williams goes out to observe
the poor defeated body in its gulfs
and grottos,[xiii] shades and shadows,
and prescribes the physic of poetry.

So imagination is lively and archaic,
seeing things in starts, in stars. Cancer is time,
it's eating us away.[xiv] It's homebody, security,
tenacious ambition. Look at the size of those
bastards, can you imagine? Slipping all over
the deck and the deck hands laughing.
What's so funny about it? Look at the time
the bastards took to get that way.

VIII. Arabesque / Autonomy

So the star shaped glial cells nourish, yes, support and insulate the neurons of the brain and spine, a glue that may bind an argument about the questions we are asking, not that we, simple laymen, simple sufferers, some say lice on the face of the planet, think much about these brain spine structures. They're simply there, doing their autonomic thing and getting small thanks in return.

Flat on our backs, in diagnostic mode, we with our big ideas of who we are and what we might be making of our lives, lie trembling as the MRI machine honks and hovers over us like a monstrous god, after which the hierophant, which is to say physician, reviews with us the bilateral growth, a shadowy shape in the occipital and temporal lobes that looks like a butterfly and is sometimes called butterfly glioma, a pretty thought but where do pretty thoughts get us here in the shadows? *Papillon.*

Some pray for deliverance, others transcendence. Some stand on the lonely mountaintop their arms outstretched. How do these structures break down is one question? What exactly can go wrong, and why shouldn't it is another. He reads the cards, the images, puts his hands lightly on our shoulder and tells us our grave fate.

But hold a minute, would you? I'm rifling through an old binder now, looking for guarantees, riffing, fumbling through receipts for HVAC and plumbing repairs, new flooring, lighting, catering, the arts of gracious living, and can find none for the greatest need of all, simply to live, perhaps to live simply if not for gods' sakes forever.

IX. Canon / Robert in the Hospital

In the hospital room, all beige and vomit green, Bob
lay listless in the standard patient bed, wearing
the standard peekaboo gown and hooked up to
the standard array of beeping machines, as his GF
Tracey, all worry and all care, said goodby. On his hip
Bob was wearing a device called Optune,[xv] wires
ascending to his shaved gauzed scalp, producing
electric tumor treating fields, TTF, to disrupt cancer
cell growth was the idea. Every sentence trailed off into
I dunno or it's weird. Sad because hadn't Bob and I written
a screenplay together, an action packed adventure that
Hollywood would not want, all about derring do and war,
for what did we know of action and adventure, till now,
when he was having the adventure of his life? By which point,
after two craniotomies, the aphasia was in full bloom and he
was texting me such texts as their in Mercy now process with
soon go die without my speech.

Yet he roused now and laughed, saying my jokes were
killing him, and tucked into the translucent veggie mess
they brought up from the bowels of the institution. No,
I said, they're keeping you alive. Potatoes au gratin,
sliced carrots, sickly iceberg lettuce, milk, and pudding
both vanilla and chocolate. Using knife for the pudding
and then a fork, he ate with relish until, staring at the crab
shaped incision above his left ear, I put a plastic spoon
in his hand.

All beige and vomit green, the hospital room and patient,
yes, and next day he attempted a jailbreak, Tracey said,
and they kept him there till they could calm him down
and return him to her care. A case of hospital delirium,
she said, a longing to escape.

X. Fugue / Up the Creek

Row, row, row your boat gently down
the stream, gliding as smoothly as you can.
Whatever creek exactly you are paddling.
Merrily. Scarily. Scantily. Ineluctably.
Row your boat, yacht, cruiser, garbage scow,
when pulling fretfully against the tide,
the pleasure seekers on the other side.
Life is but a dream.

XI. Arabesque / Raison d'Être

Forty five point two percent of malignant primary brain and CNS tumors are GBMs. Men have a slightly higher risk, though all ages and genders are affected. Make that afflicted. Biopsy and tumor debulking with post op adjuvant radio therapy and chemo via temozolomide are the most common treatments. No universal restrictions on activity are indicated. Sit down, physician, and heal thyself. Talk to the patients, set up a plan for treatment and recovery, if any. In many circumstances, physical therapy and/or rehab are extremely beneficial and may reduce risk of deep venous thrombosis. Seizures may prevent patients from driving, it's true. Talk to them, certainly, in their own language. You might discuss, for example, the lack of guarantees, the unlikelihood of survival, the good times they had when they were twenty years old and immortal, the time it will take their survivors to recover and the meds the survivors require simply to make it through the day. And, oh yes, if they're esthetically inclined and like pretty things on the wall or floor, the difference if any between objet d'art and raison d'être.

XII. Canon / Teresa's Loquacity

We met at a wine tasting, and from the start she was
chatty and genial and liked just about all the wines,
whether chardonnay or cabaret or the Merryvale pinot
noir with its dark fruit, bracing acidity, velvet touch,
its perfect weight and long evolving finish. So we began
a round of progressive dinners, going from one house
to another, testing food and wine and each other's company.

As the nights wore on, Tee became more loquacious,
until at times it became obnoxious, this birdlike piping
about nothing of interest to anyone besides herself.
At the bottom of the bottle at a wine tasting, was she
trying to get to the bottom of herself? Her talk seemed
to require no talk back. Was she circling, buzzard like,
some dead thing she couldn't quite put her beak on?

May the gods if any have
mercy on your body and
your soul, Teresa. Divorced
from husband, having
problems with your kids,
you have breathed your last
now, and may we embrace
you in the spirit of shared
suffering? Presumptuous
and fretful questions
certainly. Or what exactly
should we say, peering
straight at you into
the light?

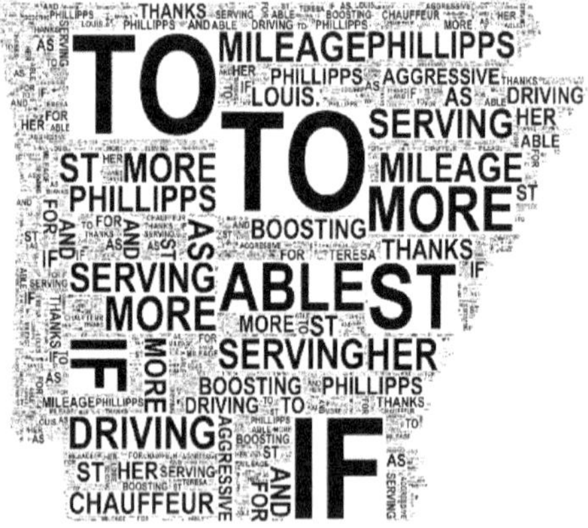

*Facebook post about chauffeuring the
author to St. Louis for a medical
procedure, 3/13/2013. Graphic via
Wordificator.*

XIII. Aria / Suffering

The stars, too, under which we
breathe and suffer, might be likened
to astrocytes, the glial structures that uphold
and support the neurons of the brain. For perhaps
it is ordained, this suffering, and endowed with a heavenly
emblem, the sign of Cancer, to remind us of what might
await us at the end, war or cancer, martial or marital
discord, whatever is torturing us, tearing us apart.
Every sentient creature suffers, for gods' sakes,
every one of us, man and beast, every mother's
son and daughter, contingent and transient.

XIV. Arabesque / Angiogenesis

The oddest thing about GBMs is how they're nourished by an ample and abnormal tumor vessel blood supply, a process called angiogenesis, regulated by proteins called angiogenic activators and inhibitors, including prions, tiny proteinaceous particles likened to viruses and viroids but having no genetic component. They said Socrates was eloquent, which he denied, and made him drink the poison because he spoke the truth.[xvi] This infiltrative blood supply can grow indefinitely, or as long as the clock ticks and tacks on any particular human being's watch. Nanomaterials might some day be taken by mouth or injection, yet how does that help us now, when we're dying, releasing antiangiogenic drugs at specific sites. Now and then, at some who knows when future date, this particular cancer cured, and we're dying of other things, gods save us. A high index of suspicion, physician, can lead to early diagnosis.

XV. Canon / Robert's Ice Cream

So a year or more later, he would still get out of the house,
Tracey's house, where he was living, every once in a while
when he was not solving jigsaw puzzles on the dining room
table or swimming laps for a half hour at a time in the
community pool or seeing the doctors. I would come for him,
spelling Tracey for a bit, and drive to the old town square,
where an ice cream truck, parked under the oaks and ashes,
vended cones, chocolate for Bob every time, and then we'd walk
around the square or to Crystal Bridges to look at the art,

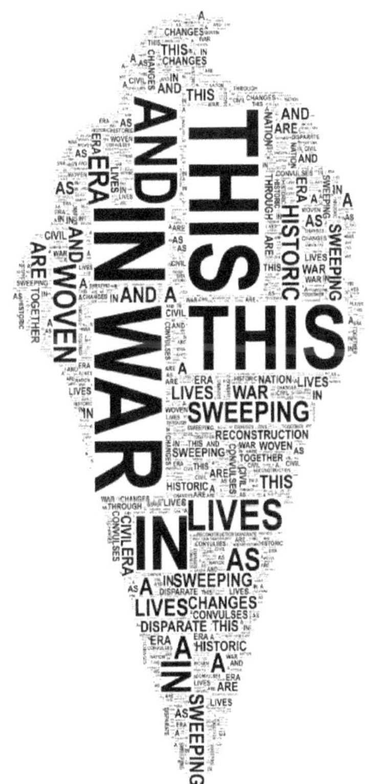

*Robert Munger, text from
opening of his novel* Scion,
Soldier, Slaves, *2022*

oneirics cut off from narrative
space and time, waiting for
something to happen, sure. I
would stand on his right side
and guide him, for by that time
the last craniotomy had robbed
him of vision in the right eye
and he wore a patch and I would
go yo ho, Bob, watch out, my
friend, and he would go I
never figured, in so many words,
it would be you of all people who
would stay by me. We had tried
that thing together, hadn't we,
that writing thing, and how did
that turn out? A year or more
later, yes, the last time I saw
him, alive, at Tracey's place, I
put my hands on his shaved,
scarred head, his face, and fed
him chocolate ice cream from
a spoon and vowed I love you,
Bob, and he said I love you too.

XVI. French Overture / Suffering and Ignorance

So our friends, our family have died, are dying
off, one by one by one, and we go on petitioning
the justice of suffering, for what do we know,
how do we know it, and how can we know more?
We carry our ideologies like millstones around
the neck. To suffer, from the Latin *sufferer,* to bear,
undergo, endure, as if we could do nothing about it.
Yet the Greeks had figured suffering heroic, Herakles
and his labors after madly killing wife and kids,
Herakles killing the Crab that Hera sent to kill him,
lighting up the heavens with the constellation Cancer.[xvii]

Suffering, long associated in the West with violating
the gods' laws, however arbitrary and inhumane
the gods may be. Is atheism, then, a consolation?
How about humanism? If we look to the ideas
of the East, we might see more clearly that every
creature suffers because we preoccupy ourselves
with our selves. That suffering is for the most part
psychological. That suffering is what the old meat
puppet does with pain. According to the Upanishads,
Dukkha, stress and suffering, is our lot in life for seeking
satisfaction from that which can never satisfy.

XVII. Arabesque / Average Survival Rate

So cancer is scary, yes? The word, the deed? The crab that clutches and devours us? We want to know how long we have to live and do we dare ask? This ain't Vegas, and the Greek ain't giving odds.[xviii] For what it's worth, one study indicates the median survival rate for adults is 14.6 months. Yet the longest survivor lived over 25 years. Rates change, as you might imagine, with each new estimate and treatment. Rather than radiotherapy and chemo, why not get in on a trial? Nothing to lose that way, right? Just six point eight percent of patients survive five years.

XVIII. Canon / Brother Dogboy

My mentor / dementor how long,
the way older siblings often are, Gerry
knew only what he knew, after all, like
the rest of us, or wanted or sought to know,
including a healthy dissent up to a point from
our parents' standard Catholic puritan dogma
about sex. He was just another dogboy, Mother said,
who art perhaps with Father even now in heaven, having
his way with the girls in the field, she said, zipping up his
pants and running away. Dogboy! she scolded and schooled
us, attention up and pants down, while the girls wept, she said, and bore
the burden. The way he ran away from his wife
of how many years for the younger, hotter one. So cancer
is a mark of divine retribution? For the Lord thy God is an angry God, he's
pissed, and has his reasons?

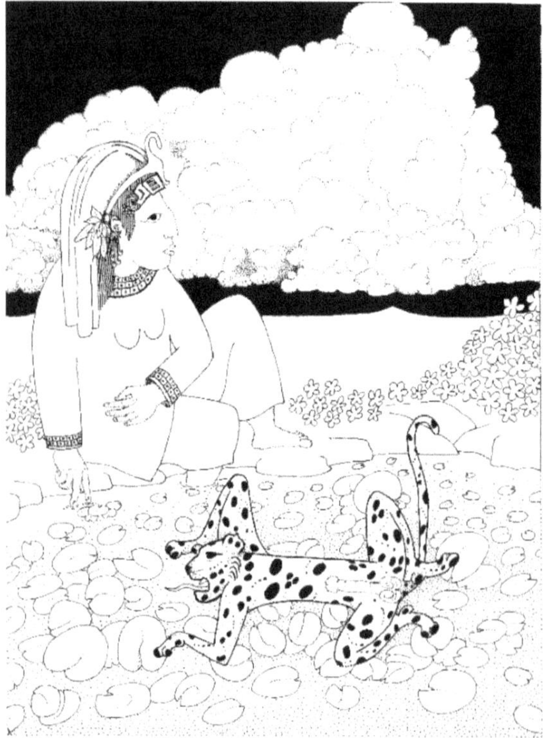

Gerry Zeck, Water Lily
Jaguar, *1994*

XIX. Dance / Crabbing

Sorry, I don't eat crab, and without a bit of mucking
about know nothing about why would I want to crab
or how is it done? Sure, they can be big bastards, but
also small, I surmise. They can feed tons of folks, those
inclined to feed thus, though others regard them as unclean
for they cannot fully process the dirt they take in, which
fills them with deadly metals and excess vitamins, or so
it's said. Or, more simply if not credibly, they have no
scales and are thus unclean. Once upon a time, long
long ago, I flew to the seminary in Ohio, for I like
my older brother Gerry before me was to study
for the priesthood, believe it or don't, but made it
just one year, until such time I became aware somehow
of the wriggling figures of women, on account of which
I too was humping the air before long like the dogboy
that I was. On the plane I was served crab and promptly
threw it up. Crab pots, I found out some time later,
rest on the bottom of the ocean and typically consist
of a wire cage about one yard square with funnel
shaped openings for the crabs to enter. The bait
is inside and the crabs are trapped in the labyrinth.
Nearly 10,700,000 tons of crustaceans, from what
I gather, were produced in a recent year, the vast
majority decapods like crabs, lobsters, shrimp,
crawfish, and prawns, with China producing
and perhaps consuming nearly half the total.
Feeding on crab, the crab feeding on us.
We dance our little jig upon the greensward
till the jig is up.

XX. Arabesque / Surprising Facts about Brain Cancer

Yes, GBMs spread by angiogenesis, rich networks of blood vessels
developing throughout the brain. Without treatment other than surgery and
radiation, survival rate, according to yet another guesstimate, is just twelve
point one months, though now there's the Optune option too, at
opportunity for the medtech industry to bill the federal government
$12,500 per month per patient. Three in ten people diagnosed with GBM
will survive two years. Men are more likely to get it than women. Ditto
people in their sixties. About 14,000 new GBM cases are diagnosed every
year in the USA. Every year for the past 30 years, the cancer has been
increasing 1.2 percent. Our chance of getting GBM is about one in
100,000, but I don't know 100,000 folks, do you? I'm no statistician, but
statisticians tell us we might know clusters? Folks and figures might be
gathered there, in the center of the bell curve and whatever it is that we
know.

XXI. Canon / Teresa's Ordeal

The thing about glioblastomas, she said, is that
they shoot out tiny tumor satellites, so even when
the tumor is removed, it's not all removed, because
these little bastards are busy setting up house
in the background. Angiogenesis, for sure.
From the outset, she said, she was striving,
and would continue to strive, for her kids' sake
if not her own to live. It was gut wrenching, she said,
to hear her adult son for one sob on the phone, so far
away, back in Arkansas, and going through his own
hell without the booze to support him and the bitch
who'd been his wife and their son. Here's some
pills, said the doctors, take 'em, which may or may
not help you straighten out your life.

Meanwhile, back in upstate New York state, the thing
about glioblastomas, she aid, is the doctors ran her
through the gamut of surgeries, chemo, radiation, sure,
the whole bloody gauntlet, and she tried to put a brave
face on it all. My address, she wrote me, is so and so
road, Hamilton, New York. are you coming to visit me?

And then she wrote no
more. Post diagnosis, she
lasted twenty two months,
longer than most, and I
never came to see her or
lived to see her take up
her pallet and walk.[xix]

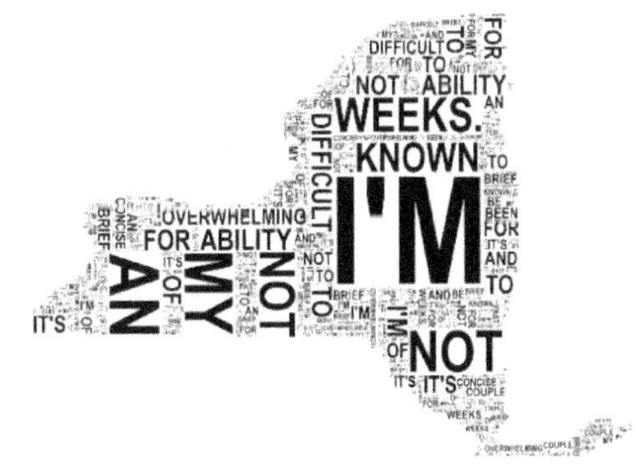

Teresa Phillipps, Facebook post, 12/1/2019.
Graphic via Wordificator

XXII. Fugue / Gerald in Hades Dream

So it wasn't I who rowed, rowed, rowed my boat
but Charon, nor gently, across the dark and roiling
stream, and there I met my brother in the underworld,
fallen wayfarer, under the aegis of Hades, the helm
of sulfurous darkness, the dark fire streaming off the god.

Brother, I implored, come back to us, as quickly
as you can. And so I prayed, in the dark, in ignorance,
come back the way you walked and looked in your glory,
not the way you looked the day that I arrived four hours
late the day you died, Columbus Day and you weren't going
anywhere, less than four months post diagnosis, and lay
there cold and motionless on the mortuary slab, and your
son Chris and I, at the corpse our station keeping, stood over
you weeping. You have a lot of work to do, I said, gripping
your forearm, so many fine lines to pursue to their end,
artist, brother, seeker, friend. Telos, remember, I said,
from the Greek *télos*.

Come back? he said, smiling, breaking my grip.
Yes, he said, if it were possible, here where everything
passes and is past. Time and time again, he said, our time
is passing, and time in passing is all we have. His eyes glowed
and told the story of impossible longing, and suddenly I fell
back and was once more in the middle of life's wood,
where I'd been walking, unenlightened, on life's
path, and blinking in the dazzling light of day.

XXIII. Arabesque / Questions Technical and Not

Even as the blood chills, my friends, we're raising funds for research, *a la recherche de temps perdu,* and what time is not lost? You can find lots of ways to get involved, for example, join in fund raising or fund walking / running /biking. Donate to the National Brain Tumor Association. Get off the couch and hop on your bike. Reach out and touch someone via social media. Look for a doctor with experience in assessment and diagnosis, knowledgeable about the latest advanced procedures. Ask herm why did three point nine percent of patients who received TAFINLAR + MEKINIST have fatal ARs, that is, Adverse Reactions? Consider can we beat brain cancer by using the eleven effective treatment strategies covered in the new report? Make it your business to know how brain cancer stem cell research is progressing, given that brain cancer stem cells drive the persistence of malignant tumors. Do you know that lymphocyte specific tyrosine kinase (Lck) might be targeted in the malignant tissue and used to prevent growth and metastasis? Finally, ask what do surgeons and other tech experts know of the inevitability of suffering and managing pain not by looking on the bright side of life or by cramming technical data up our credulous posteriors?

XXIV. Canon / Gerald RIP

He is gone, gone where the good and the bad alike go.
Gone with no ghost of himself remaining I can see
but what I see on the walls of my home study,
my scuttling brain borne up against the darkest day
by an array of his line drawings, mystic, magic,
yearning, cloudscape and landscape, a Mayan rain
god for example and Tanda bursting with eggs,
Tanda's pen inviting us to create, a sculptor
chiseling an inscription in the clouds.

Ab ovo, brother, we are born and then we die, marveling, nourishing,
searching, being. *Ave, frater, atque vale.*[xx]

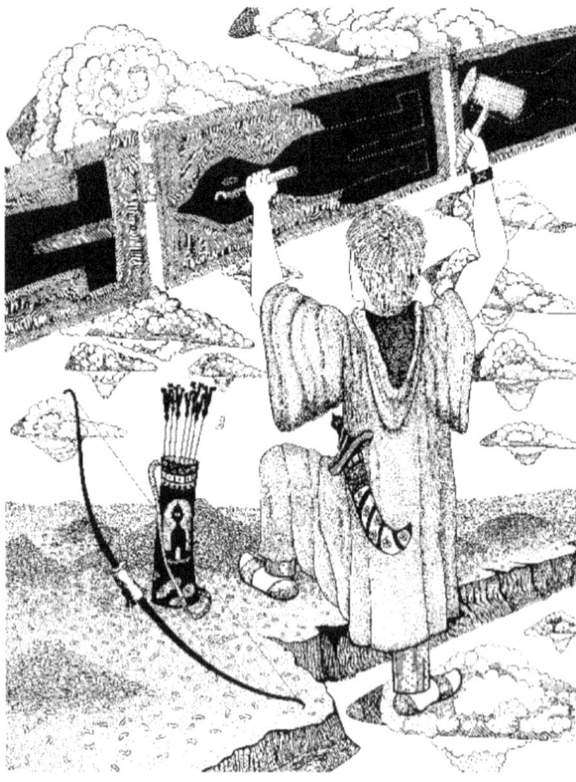

Gerry Zeck, Clouds, *with inscription "The clouds pass and the man does his work and all beings flow into their form," ND.*

XXV. Aria / Another Point of View

Yes, we try to get it
through our heads. Our
thick occipitals and minds
bogged down by the idea of
suffering, by the fact of suffering,
by the question of fairness. Are they
passing out of this life, these other animals,
so that we might stay? The mind itself, like a
dying star, blinking on and off, irradiates our doubts.
Star of wonder, star of night, where are the answers burning
bright? The glory if any and the resurrection? Rising in
the east and setting in the west, looking for a savior
to save us from ourselves, from the all too easy
answers, even as the meat puppet cowers in
the corner. Suffering, it's said, is a domain
of ironies through which we might be
enlightened, lightened, ascend.
Loaves and fishes indeed. Crabs
and butterflies. Sorrow and delusion,
say the Upanishads, come to the ignorant.
When we are dead, is it possible we are not
dead, can we get this through our heads, but
transposed, migrated from one body to another?
Imagine how boring it would be to be in the same
place in the same time forever, placid, unchanging.
Is that what you would call paradise? Frankly,
can I be frank here, what do I know and do we
have a choice in the matter? What do these
changes have to do with choice?

XXVI. Arabesque / Tumor Suppression

A number of aberrations are common to all cancers, and all patients it may be, including the silencing of Tumor Suppressing Genes, a driving event in the oncogenic process and the silencing of hope. With this in mind, great efforts have been made to develop small molecules aimed at the restoration of TSGs. In patients with High Grade Gliomas, epigenetic silencing of the MGMT enzyme and other jargon may be associated with improved survival rates.

XXVII. Canon / Robert's New Year Day

He died this last New Year's Day and so found
a way out of suffering, a new life in the stars,
in the constellation Cancer, it could be: just
590 light years up and away, shining however
faintly. And shouldn't we be looking up more
constantly? One of twelve zodiac constellations,
a clock by which we might learn at last to tell time
and defy it. Creator by birth and architect by vocation,
Bob designed buildings even if he could not quite, any
more than you or I, design an entire life. Closing our eyes
on the mountaintop, blotting out the city's pollutions,
reaching out our arms to empty or not empty space,
balanced for a moment with a peculiar grace, allowed
this gesture for a moment, we accede.

*Robert Munger, text from his 2011
novel* The Charette Legacy,
*published under the pseudonym
John Highsmith Adams. Graphic
via Wordificator*

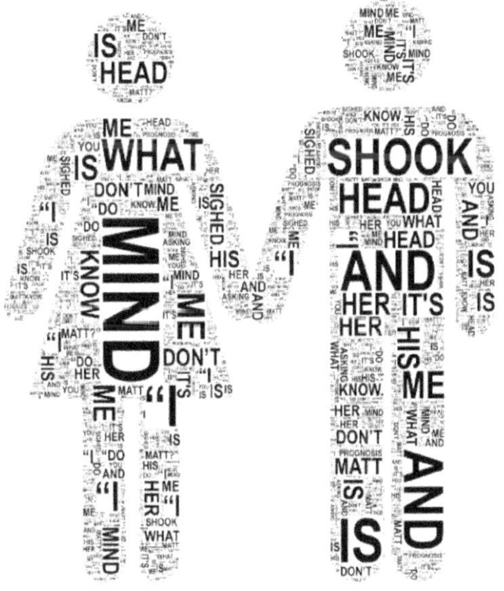

XXVIII. Fugue / Teresa's Dream

And so the days blazed by in glory
and so it was vouchsafed that Teresa
came to me one night in dream,
and I dreamed that the dream
text itself spellbound and confounded
me, *timor mortis conturbat me,*[xxi]
a little Latin goes a long long
way and less Greek, for Tee
had been texting all her friends
but me, I felt guilty and reached
out my hands to her shade
imploringly, her dim figure,
waveringly, and said, Teresa,
talk to me now (say twenty
five words or fewer, make
them last). And at that instant
she flared like a spit of fire
and vanished suddenly.
If spirits can be said to exist,
mysteriously. And went down
to dark Avernus.

XXIX. Arabesque / Life Is Short

Does it come down finally to the fact that life is short? And that while art, including dance, song, love, and poetry, is often long, or said to be, our kisses burning hot and bright,[xxii] then what? Then what? That poetry and philosophy may be more valuable than medicine? That to die is far different from what anyone supposed, and luckier?[xxiii] That reading the tech lit may make us smarter, in a narrow sense, but a narrow sense is not what is needed at this hour? That pain is a given, in other words, but suffering is optional? That suffering may be part of craving, and what do we crave, now and at the hour of our death, amen, we weak and pitiable human creatures?

XXX. Quodlibet

Were you too raised a believer?[xxiv] Did you too go up
to the altar of God, the God that gave joy to youth,[xxv]
the God that supplied benevolent loaves and fishes
to the multitudes assembled on the hillside hungry
for the word, a story that we might choose to believe
or not? Faithful or heathen or humanist, when we
encounter these questions of suffering and justice,
huddling and trembling in our boots or slippers,
do we cry out from the depths? When a friend
is strapped to the altar, an oblation, and the knife
descends, is suffering mandated? Whose choice?
Whose chance? So where is it written and who says
it's fair that Gerald and Teresa and Robert, or any
of the faceless countless others afflicted each year
are the ones to be sacrificed? Who says? And who
gainsays the gesture, touch, and glance, the glory
of the song and dance as long as they lasted and do last?

Aria / Theme & Glory

Yes, let the astrocytes,
the star shapes in our brains,
point the way we are going, every
last mother's son and daughter transient,
contingent, touching, shining, suffering. The loaves
and fishes multiplied, the crab cakes distributed, animal,
anima, telos, end. The texts, well woven or not, technical or
not, discerned. Let us row our boats, rejoice, life is such
a dream. The sun, our star, is shining, yes. Emerge,
brothers, sisters, from the cave. Live as long
and as fiercely as you can in the light.

Endnotes

[i] Stephen Batchelor, *Confessions of a Buddhist Atheist,* quoted in Derek Beres, https://bigthink.com/articles/is-suffering-necessary-for-the-spiritual-life.

[ii] From Stevens' collection *The Auroras of Autumn* (1950). Reprinted online at https://billcollinsenglish.com/Ordinary EveningHaven.html.

[iii] From Crane's first poem collection, *White Buildings* (1926). Reprinted online in many places, including https://allpoetry. com/Repose-Of-Rivers. The first aria in Bach's Variations is in the form of a sarabande, a slow Spanish dance in 3/4 time.

[iv] See https://www.tvo.org/transcript/005584/interview-carl-sagan.

[v] See https://en.wikipedia.org/wiki/Goldberg_Variations.

[vi] See the website of the Bach Museum in Leipzig, Germany at https://www.bachmuseumleipzig.de/sites/ default/files/ u8809/ 2024_6_Goldberg Variations.pdf. Also very helpful in understanding the structure and forms of Bach's masterpiece are https://www.wikiwand.com/en/articles/Goldberg_ Variations and https://www.wikiwand.com/en/articles/ Ralph_Kirkpatrick.

[vii] The first section of Bach's "Goldberg Variations," the aria, is "a sarabande, one of the dances common to the baroque suite. In Bach's solo works for harpsichord, violin, and cello, it is the most expressive movement of the suite, often contemplative and tender." Charlotte Nediger, https://tafelmusik.org/explore- baroque/articles/behind-musik-bach-goldberg-variations/.

[viii] German for not true, isn't it so? Equivalent to French *n'est pas.*

[ix] See www.wordificator.com.

[x] This image comes from an episode of *The Deadliest Catch,* I believe. See https://en.wikipedia.org/wiki/Deadliest_Catch. The crab has long been associated with cancer, "the oldest and most pervasive zoomorphic image of cancer," according to A. Skuse, "Constructions of Cancer in Early Modern England: Ravenous Natures," https://www.

ncbi.nlm.nih.gov/books/ NBK547261/.

[xi] In Plato's allegory of the cave, people are chained to the cave walls and mistake shadows for reality. See https://en/wikipedia.org/wiki/Allegory_of_the_cave.

[xii] Henry Miller, *Tropic of Cancer,* 1934, first page of the novel.

[xiii] See https://www.poetryfoundation.org/poets/william-carlos-williams. William Carlos Williams was one of the great American modernist poets of the first half of the 20th century and a practicing medical doctor. He would sometimes write out poems on prescription pads.

[xiv] Henry Miller again, as in note xii above.

[xv] The Optune is "a wearable, portable, FDA-approved glioblastoma (GBM) treatment for adult patients aged 22 years or older. It works by creating Tumor Treating Fields (TTF), which are electric fields that can slow down or stop GBM cancer division," https://www.optunegio.com/.

[xvi] In Plato, *The Apology,* Socrates says about his accusers, "they have hardly spoken a word of truth. But many as their falsehoods were, there was one of them which quite amazed me—I mean when they told you to be upon your guard, and not to let yourselves be deceived by the force of my eloquence. They ought to have been ashamed of saying this, because they were sure to be detected as soon as I opened my lips and displayed my deficiency; they certainly did appear to be most shameless in saying this, unless by the force of eloquence they mean the force of truth…." https://chs.harvard.edu/primary-source/ plato-the-apology-of-socrates-sb/.

[xvii] See https://www.britannica.com/topic/Heracles: "Heracles' life was marred by intense guilt and suffering, largely stemming from the madness inflicted upon him by Hera. In a fit of rage, he killed his wife and children, an act that haunted him for the rest of his life. This tragedy highlights the psychological burden he carried, shaping his character and motivating his quest for redemption. See also https://www.theoi.com/ Ther/Karkinos.html: "Karkinos (Carcinus) was a giant crab which came to the aid of the Hydra in its battle with Herakles [Hercules] at Lerna. The hero crushed it beneath his foot but as a reward for its service the goddess Hera placed it amongst the stars as the constellation Cancer." Consider

also "Cancer the Crab in the Zodiac," https: www.liveabout.com/cancer-the- crab-zodiac-signs-206380.

[xviii] James George Snyder Sr., known popularly as Jimmy the Greek, 1918–1996, sports commentator and bookie. See https://en.wikipedia.org/wiki/Jimmy_Snyder_(sports_ commentator).

[xix] John 5:8. See https://biblehub.com/john/5-8.htm.

[xx] *Ab ovo,* from the egg, at the start. *Ave, frater, atque vale:* Hail, brother, and farewell, from an elegy by the Roman poet Catullus to his dead brother. See https://www.pantheonpoets. com/poems/catulluss-farewell-to-his-brother/.

[xxi] *Timor mortis conturbat me:* the fear of death confounds me. For one example of this medieval Latin refrain, see https:// genius. com/Medival-bbes-timor-mortis-conturbat-me-lyrics.

[xxii] I'm thinking here of Franz Lehar's operetta *Giuditta,* "Meine Lippen Sie Küssen So Heiss" ("My Lips They Kiss So Hot"). For an especially fun and fiery rendition of the song, see Anna Netrebko at https://www.youtube.com/watch?v=tcidmfVkc10.

[xxiii] Walt Whitman, *Song of Myself,* part 6: https://www. poetryfoundation.org/poems/45477/ song-of-myself-1892-version.

[xxiv] Quodlibet: according to Merriam-Webster, this musical term, used by Bach for this section of the *Goldberg Variations,* signifies a couple of things: first, "a whimsical combination of familiar melodies or texts," and second, more to the point here, "a philosophical or theological point proposed for disputation." https://www.merriam-webster.com/dictionary/quodlibet.

[xxv] Douay-Rheims Version, Psalms 43:4. These are also the beginning words of the Catholic mass: I will go up to the altar of God, to God who gives joy to my youth. See https://biblehub. com/ catholic/psalms/43-4.htm.